◆

The making of an
EFFICIENT
PHYSICIAN

◆

By
Sherry Anderson Delio, MPA, HSA
&
George Hein, ABC, APR

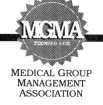

MEDICAL GROUP
MANAGEMENT
ASSOCIATION

Medical Group Management Association (MGMA) publications are intended to provide current and accurate information and are designed to assist readers in becoming more familiar with the subject matter covered. Such publications are distributed with the understanding that MGMA does not render any legal, accounting or other professional advice that may be construed as specifically applicable to individual situations. No representation or warranties are made concerning the application of legal or other principles discussed by the author to any specific fact situation, nor is any prediction made concerning how any particular judge, government official or other person who will interpret or apply such principles. Specific factual situations should be discussed with professional advisors.

◆

Table of contents

◆

Table of contents

◆

Acknowledgments

◆

All the material in this book was developed from observations of hundreds of physicians' practices. Without the kindness, perceptiveness and insight of the people working in the physicians' office as well as the managers, supervisors and administrators, none of this would have been possible.

We also would like to thank the physicians that were kind enough to let us spend time following them throughout their days with a stop watch. It is not easy to have someone record every move you make. It shows how committed these physicians were to improving patient care.

We would like to thank all the patients that sat through the focus groups, answered surveys and were open and honest with us about the care they expected.

A big thank you to Dr. Melvin Freeman for his help with the title.

And finally, a special thanks to the staff members at MGMA for making the publication of this book possible: **Fred E. Graham II, PhD, FACMPE**, Senior Associate Executive Director; **Dennis L. Barnhardt, APR**, Director of Communications; **Barbara U. Hamilton, MA**, Library Resource Center Director; **Brenda Hull**, Communications Project Manager; **Cynthia Kiyotake**, Librarian; **Stephanie Wyllyamz**, Communications Specialist; and **Ellie Cox**, Communications Administrative Secretary.

◆

Foreword

◆

The health care industry faces tremendous challenges in the years ahead. We continue to confront clinical challenges as we strive to best serve our patients. The delivery of medicine has become increasingly complex, and now faces unprecedented limitations on resource utilization. We see a better educated, better informed patient population with high expectations.

Are we meeting our patients' needs? Are we optimizing value by providing levels of quality and service that meet the high standards our medical profession and the health care industry sets for itself? These are important questions that we all must ask ourselves if we are to chart a successful course for the future. As we attempt to affirm that we are indeed meeting the expectations set by our patients, our purchasers, and ourselves, we often come face-to-face with the need to change.

All too often we become insular, set in our ways — we resist change. At Virginia Mason Medical Center, we've been fortunate to have Sherry Delio and George Hein as part of our staff, challenging our preconceived notions. Delio has successfully worked with clinicians in all specialties. Initial skepticism amongst our clinicians ("An efficiency expert? No way!") has given way to acceptance and a long waiting list of primary care and specialty departments requesting and eagerly awaiting review by our practice management program led by Delio. As a result of these reviews, productivity and patient, physician and staff satisfaction all have been enhanced.

In *The Making of an Efficient Physician*, Delio and Hein present us with an easy-to-read manual for understanding our daily work life and provide tools and a method for improvement. The principles are simple, logical and utilize many of the basic tenets of quality improvement. The approach is "customer driven" and relies heavily on data, rather than anecdote. This has tremendous appeal for physicians as we pride ourselves on making data-driven decisions. Delio and Hein start with "observation" and provide through their continuous stopwatch study methods, information that provides a framework for the "six guiding principles." These principles, when fully enacted by departments at Virginia Mason Medical Center, have resulted in major improvements in efficiency, service and satisfaction.

It is important to keep in mind that reduction in resource utilization may seemingly reduce costs, but sometimes at the expense of quality and customer satisfaction. The authors understand this well as they delineate what is truly possible as we improve efficiency. Eliminating variation, and thereby enhancing predictability for patients and staff, can be extremely powerful. Applying resources proportional to volume and methods for doing so are essential. Appropriate task distribution, facilitating physicians doing work that is truly "physician work," nurses doing work that takes advantage of their clinical expertise, and appropriately utilizing staff in all areas, leads to enhanced performance. The importance of this highly developed team interdependency cannot be overstated.

Change inevitably results in varying levels of acceptance. This certainly is true for physicians and medical groups. The authors give us a blueprint for understanding that which we do every day. The opportunities and challenges are immense, and Sherry Delio and George Hein have provided us with tools to truly delight our customers and ourselves.

Gary S. Kaplan, M.D.
Chief Division of Satellites
Virginia Mason Medical Center

♦

Chapter 1
Introduction

♦

Make your practice the best

This book is a down-to-earth guide to running an efficient medical practice.

On the following pages, you will find out exactly how to set up and run a well-oiled practice — or how to revamp and improve a chaotic one. If you follow the recommendations and guidelines here, your practice can be one of the best anywhere.

In an era of proposed health care reform, narrowing profit margins and increased competition, making a practice more efficient is a powerful tool for coping with the change. There may be much in the health care environment that you cannot alter; however, you do have the ability to make your own practice strong, well-managed and profitable.

This book shows you how. While it may look disarmingly simple, it cuts to the core of an efficient practice. You will discover clear, proactive steps — strategies you can put into practice today. Within several months, you can be using every technique in this book.

Furthermore, it includes samples of forms that you need. These are copyright free and adaptable for your use.

Use this as a survival manual for managers, physicians and staff

When you have finished this book, you will discover that you have completed a crash-course in practice survival skills. Quite simply, that means you will learn to cut out wasted time and effort, work efficiently and create an environment in which physicians can see more patients with less stress. This contributes to genuine value offered to your patients and the insurance companies and others that pay the claims.

When we talk about value, we are talking about providing appropriate care that leads to quality outcomes — all delivered in the context of excellent service and offered at a reasonable price. By using the key management principles in this book, you can immediately enhance patient care by improving the operational systems that support the patient-physician interaction.

In years of consulting with physicians, one of the most common concerns we hear is: If I could spend more time taking care of patients and less time on paperwork, I'd be happy.

This book meets both those goals. It shows managers how to create a practice operation based on solid systems, open communication, time-efficient protocols and a genuine concern for patient, physician and staff satisfaction.

As a result, physicians can see more patients in a more orderly, relaxed way. The practice also will gain a reputation among both patients and payers as being a place of true value — the key competitive advantage for the next decade.

Tap the expertise of professionals with decades of experience

The gems you will discover in this book are gleaned from decades of on-the-job practice experience. The author's experience ranges from analyzing one-physician offices to re-engineering a 400-provider multispecialty clinic.

As a practice management consultant, Sherry Delio has spent the past decade observing and conducting time-and-motion studies of hundreds of medical practices. She has developed, tested, refined and perfected dozens of techniques and systems for achieving maximum productivity with the least amount of effort. She has analyzed thousands of patient surveys and participated in many patient focus groups. Delio is a sought-after national speaker on practice management with a proven track record for turning around both large and small medical practices.

Co-author George Hein is one of a handful of communicators fully accredited by both International Association of Business Communicators (IABC) and Public Relations Society of America (PRSA). He has worked in health care communications both at the corporate level and within hospitals. While at Adventist Health System, he helped develop one of the first nationally used nurse phone consulting programs and more recently helped plan one of the first interactive patient communication systems to operate on the Internet, a network of computers worldwide ranging from individual users to large educational, corporate or governmental institutions.

Together, this team shares what they have learned about methods for building a practice that runs smoothly, satisfies patients and retains staff.

So why not get started? Set aside 90 minutes — the approximate time it will take you to zoom through this book.

◆

Chapter 2

A chaotic medical practice

◆

The following fictitious case illustrates behavior we have witnessed during our studies. Few practices are as chaotic as Dr. Frazzle's practice. Many of these problems however, occur in numerous practices. Inefficient systems compromise quality patient care in all systems whether you are 100 percent managed care or still heavily fee-for-service.

Lack of a clear understanding of how physicians practice often results in systems that inhibit rather than enhance physician's productivity and customer service, which are essential in an efficient, effective medical practice.

First, let's visit the practice of Dr. Frazzle and see how well-intentioned activities can eat away at a physician's time and be misinterpreted by the patient.

Ms. Ann Ackney arrives for her 8:30 a.m. appointment. Rudy, the receptionist, slides back the window and greets her with a curt, "What is your name?"

"Ann Ackney," states Ann.

"I can't find your chart; what other name do you go by?" says Rudy indifferently.

"No other name," says Ann.

"Dr. Frazzle isn't here yet; go sit down," says Rudy as she closes the window and continues to socialize with her co-workers.

Ms. Ackney waits until 9:15 a.m. and then decides to ask how much longer she must wait. Rudy shoots a glare at her and says, "How should I know when he will return to the office? He's always late." Ms. Ackney returns to her chair and decides she will wait only 15 minutes more.

Right at 9:30 a.m., Dr. Frazzle walks through the door and greets Ms. Ackney. He walks her back to the exam room, apologizing the entire way. After instructing her to put on the gown, he leaves the exam room and enters his office. His "in" box is full of telephone messages that he returns before seeing Ms. Ackney.

Dr. Frazzle hangs up the telephone. It is now 10 a.m. Again, the first thing he does when he enters the room is apologize for being late, explaining that he was on the telephone with a very sick patient.

Because he does not have Ms. Ackney's chart, he apologizes for the missing chart and asks the patient to review her history for him. She states that she never heard back about the test results from her last visit.

Dr. Frazzle leaves the room to ask Bertha, his back-office support staff member, to track down the results of the previous tests. The only copy of the test results is in the lost medical record, so Bertha calls the lab. When she finally gets the results, she has to interrupt Dr. Frazzle again to give them to him.

Dr. Frazzle decides he needs to do a procedure, so he reaches into the cupboard for some supplies; of course, they are out of stock. As his frustration level increases, he excuses himself from Ms. Ackney and retrieves the needed supplies.

He returns with the supplies, completes the procedure and reviews the diagnosis and treatment plan with Ms. Ackney. Dr. Frazzle leaves the room while she is dressing. He stands behind Bertha, waiting for her to get off the telephone. Bertha sees Dr. Frazzle, puts the caller on hold and listens to Dr. Frazzle shout out his orders for Ms. Ackney. He then enters his second patient's exam room — 90 minutes late.

Ms. Ackney leaves the exam room and waits for Bertha to end her telephone conversation. The two discuss Dr. Frazzle's orders before Ann leaves. When she gets to the elevator, she remembers that Dr. Frazzle said he was going to start her on a new medication; however, he never gave her the prescription. She returns to the office and tells Rudy what has happened.

Rudy asks her to sit down as she talks to Bertha. Dr. Frazzle is with another patient, so Bertha interrupts Dr. Frazzle to get the prescription. She finally takes it out to Ms. Ackney.

Ann proceeds to the lab to have her blood drawn. Dr. Frazzle said he would call her the next day with the results. She is anxious and worries that Dr. Frazzle may again forget to call her with the results of her tests. She is losing confidence in Dr. Frazzle, not because of his lack of expertise, but because of his chaotic practice.

When Ann arrives at the pharmacy, the pharmacist tells her he cannot interpret the prescription and has to call Dr. Frazzle's office. Ann waits again.

Back at the office, Bertha again interrupts Dr. Frazzle to take the telephone call from the pharmacy. His frustration level increases. He shouts the order to the pharmacist with a few unkind words.

Once Ann is home she forgets Dr. Frazzle's instructions about what she could and could not eat. He told her to call back if she had any questions — so she does. Rudy answers the telephone and puts Ms. Ackney on hold before she has a chance to speak. After several minutes, Rudy answers the call again, takes the message and hangs up the telephone. Ann waits two hours and hears nothing from the doctor, so she calls again. This time Rudy seems irritated that she is calling a second time. Rudy tells her that Dr. Frazzle is busy and will call her back when he has time. Offended by her tone, Ann hangs up and feels angry at Dr. Frazzle. Her confidence is waning.

At 7 p.m. Dr. Frazzle finishes with his last patient. He walks into his office and sees a pile of charts that he needs to dictate and an "in" box full of telephone messages and mail. He saw 14 patients today — but it seemed like 25. An exhausted Dr. Frazzle feels he is losing control of his practice.

"Is it worth it?" he wonders.

As you can see from this fictitious case study, hard work and devotion alone do not equal a well-run practice.

While we realize not all days go like this day with Dr. Frazzle, too often we are seeing care compromised because of the increased frustration in the work place. Lack of organization and teamwork leaves patients questioning the competence of their physicians.

The following 11 chapters will give you helpful hints and guidance for turning chaos into an organized, efficient medical practice. Practice managers must develop systems that support the physician/patient interaction. It is imperative that the entire team, as well as leadership, focuses on quality care as perceived by the patient.

◆

Chapter 3

Six guiding principles

◆

What we can learn from Dr. Frazzle

His practice is what we call a "reactive" practice. When a problem or situation occurs, both the support staff and Dr. Frazzle fly into a hyperactive mode and react to the situation, using increased energy and resources. Reactive practices create little job satisfaction and a great deal of patient dissatisfaction.

"Proactive" practices, on the other hand, create job satisfaction, decrease stress levels in the work place and increase patient satisfaction.

Physicians cannot create a proactive environment alone. It takes leadership that understands the operational needs of both the patient and physician to guide the development of systems to support a proactive approach to patient care.

Dr. Frazzle's practice lacks leadership, teamwork, clarity and planning. Dr. Frazzle's vision for his practice is not clear.

If Dr. Frazzle could take the time to analyze his practice and articulate his vision for his practice, his support staff could embrace his vision. This illustration clearly shows that his support staff members do not take responsibility for their jobs or feel part of his vision.

Developing systems based on the following guiding principles could help Dr. Frazzle actually increase his volume of patients per day while gaining control of his practice.

We often hear people say that the objective of managed care is to see fewer patients not more. While it is true you do not want to use health care resources unnecessarily, you do want to be able to manage the care of a larger population of patients efficiently. The number of patients you are responsible for caring for will determine your allocation of health care dollars. Primary care physician's income will most likely be related to the number of patients they are responsible for managing. This is often referred to as their panel size. As you can see, it will be important in both the managed care environment and the fee-for-service environment, that physicians care for a maximum number of patients per day. It is important to develop a framework for a high volume practice. Six guiding principles are the basis for our framework.

Let these principles guide your practice

Guiding principles are like road maps that keep everyone moving in the appropriate direction. If you plan to drive from Seattle to Miami, there are many ways you can choose to get there. However, if your directions tell you to go through Chicago and Washington, D.C., you will take a very different route than if you must go through Los Angeles. Guiding principles take you on the most efficient, effective route to attain your vision.

Here are the six practice management guiding principles used in our studies:

- making a time commitment;

- balancing work loads;

- decreasing unnecessary variation;

- distributing tasks appropriately;

- creating a team — interdependency; and

- allocating resources by volume of work.

This proactive approach focuses on planning ahead — anticipating what may happen. The following is a short overview of each practice management guiding principle. You will read about each principle more completely in later chapters.

The first guiding principle is making a time commitment. Everyone on the health care team must commit to value-oriented care. Commitment relates to the amount of time and effort dedicated to seeing patients. Patients value communication with their physicians.

The second is balancing work loads. A balanced patient schedule improves service levels, reduces stress and creates satisfied patients.

Compliance and consistency improve with standardization. The third guiding principle focuses on decreasing unnecessary variation. Consistency enhances a patient's confidence in the system.

The fourth principle is distributing tasks appropriately. The rule of thumb we use is to delegate to the lowest skill-level person who can safely and legally perform a task. This increases job satisfaction and decreases costs. It also frees up the physician to spend more time with patients.

Creating a team-interdependency is the fifth principle. Many management texts document the advantages of teamwork in the work place. People working in teams seem to perform more effectively than people working in isolation.

The sixth is allocating resources by volume of work. A high-volume practice needs both more space and support staff than a practice with lower volumes. A typical allocation of resources per physician is one office, two exam rooms and one support staff. This is not always appropriate and often creates barriers for high-volume physicians.

Before we focus on the details of the practice management guiding principles, we first must discuss in the next two chapters the importance of mission statements and patient expectations.

◆

Chapter 4

Best value in town

◆

Create a mission statement

In our practice management program, most physicians chose a mission statement based on being "the best value in town" where value equals excellent service plus appropriate care with quality outcomes at a reasonable cost. When everyone focuses on value, they will better understand what is most important to the practice — customer service, appropriate care, quality outcomes and costs. Behaviors that do not enhance the mission statement are not appropriate.

Reflecting back on Dr. Frazzle, we can see that many of the behaviors demonstrated in the illustration would not meet the expectations of this mission statement. Why are you in business?

If you want to build a successful practice, you must first analyze where you are going and how you will get there. Building a successful practice requires input and cooperation from many people. First, however, you must understand your patient's needs. Too often physicians build practices based on their own perceptions. It is the patient's perceptions that are most important. The only way you will know your patients' needs and desires is to ask them.

The first step in building a successful practice is to establish a mission statement. A mission statement explains your reason for existing as a practice in clear, concise, simple terms.

A well-written, thoughtfully crafted mission statement can be the basis for evaluating all aspects of your business.

The process of arriving at a mission statement is sometimes as important as the end product. As part of the process, answer the following questions:

• Who do we intend to serve?

- Why should our targeted group select us over another practice?

- What do we value?

- How do we conduct our business? and

- What will we do better than anyone else?

The process of asking these questions — especially as a group — can lead to good discussions about your practice's goals, approach to patient care and distinctive place in the marketplace. Make sure all physicians in the group, as well as management and staff, agree on the mission.

As you are developing a mission statement, invite the entire staff to participate. Solicit new ideas. Foster a sense of involvement.

To initiate the discussion, you might say, "We want to condense into one or two sentences who we are and what we hope to accomplish."

A good mission statement often includes the following:

- who you plan to serve;

- what geographic area you will cover;

- what range of services you will offer;

- what your commitment to service will be;

- what your commitment to value will be; and

- how you will resolve disputes.

One clinic printed its mission statement on every appointment card. It began, "Our pledge to you, our patients..." The pledge explained what patients could routinely expect from the practice. It included the clinic's commitment to patient confidentiality, fair pricing, full disclosure and same-day appointments, when needed.

Mission statements sometimes seem exasperatingly difficult to write; like trying to cram an elephant into a test tube, there seems to be too much to say in a few short sentences.

If that happens, do not focus too heavily on the writing of the mission statement; instead think about the goals of the practice. When you clearly think through your goals, the words themselves will come easily enough.

Here is an example:

"Our mission is to provide timely, appropriate and cost-effective health care to patients who require our specialty services and to provide treatment that leads to the best outcomes in a friendly, professional, patient-focused setting."

One large clinic posted the mission statement in the lobby after every employee signed it. It made a dramatic point of entry and gave a powerful message of commitment to each patient who entered.

Too often, mission statements emerge as cold, clinical, passionless platitudes. A mission statement should have heart, soul, zest, vitality — even humor. It should mirror the personality of the office.

Here are a few more ideas about mission statements:

- **Date them and revisit them annually**. Ask your group, "Are we really achieving this mission?" If the answer is yes, celebrate. If the answer is no, either revise your mission statement or change your practice to match the objective;

- **Post the mission statement**. Put it where your patients can see it. This helps make you accountable to the people for whom you work — your patients. Seeing it on the wall also is an ever-present reminder of your value system;

- **Make it part of new-staff orientation**. Show them the mission statement. Explain how you wrote it. Talk about why you included various aspects in the mission statement; and

- **Tie key activities to the mission statement**. Use it as a road map for planning and a source of evaluating projects.

Once you have written your mission statement, ask your patients about their expectations, needs and desires and make sure your mission statement will allow you to meet their needs.

◆

Chapter 5

Seeing your practice through your patients' eyes

◆

Identify patient expectations

Let's put first things first and start with patients: the reason your medical practice exists. Ultimately, patients help you succeed or fail. Successful practices build their systems based on the desires and needs of their patients.

We recommend two different approaches to identify patients' expectations. The first approach is to write a patient satisfaction survey. Surveys help identify areas of concern to patients. The second approach is to conduct patient focus groups, which give us even more direct input about patients' expectations. Focus groups take more time, but there is no substitute for talking directly with patients.

Sound utterly simple?

It is. Somehow, in the hubbub of setting up a practice, hiring staff and developing systems, you easily can overlook the patients interests. Also, while scurrying from exam room to exam room, physicians easily can lose sight of the singular impression each patient takes away from his or her visit.

Luckily, patient's expectations are modest, indeed. A positive attitude sometimes can compensate for lack of organization. A warm smile and helpful attitude will ease most any situation.

The practice team who knows what their patients want and then meet, or exceed, those desires will have a growing, satisfied patient base.

We have compiled a patient wish list from our patient satisfaction surveys and focus groups. Meeting each of these requests is easily achievable.

The importance of names

The most beautiful word in a person's language is his or her own name. Calling a person by name immediately shows recognition, respect and concern. Encourage every member of the team to use people's names.

Similarly, patients like to know with whom they are dealing. Every staff member should wear a badge with his or her name and title. Patients often believe they are speaking to a registered nurse when, in fact, they are talking to a clerical support person. They also sometimes believe they are talking with a physician when they are talking with a physician's assistant.

Appropriate scheduling

Patients' expectations are very clear as to the length of time they are willing to wait when they call for an appointment. While many patients tell us they will wait a long time to see a particular physician, they do not think it is acceptable.

If a patient calls with an emergency, tell him or her immediately to call 911. If the patient has an urgent health concern, schedule him or her within 24 hours. Schedule patients with chief complaints within four days. A two-week wait for other routine appointments generally is acceptable.

Proper waiting area

Patients expect clean and neat waiting areas. Patients appreciate chairs that they easily can get in and out of. We often hear patients complain about outdated reading material in waiting rooms.

Communicating about delays

Patients will wait patiently for about 15 minutes. If the wait is longer than that, please tell the patient why.

Be honest and patients usually will be understanding, especially if you are dealing with an emergency or an especially difficult case.

Exam room protocol for physicians

- **Enter the exam room prepared**. Look at the chart before entering the room. Introduce yourself to the patient. Many patients say they find it disconcerting when their physician seems to be fumbling through their charts looking for facts or their name;

- **Review the history**. This is where a one-page summary sheet of the patient's problems, treatments and medications will save physicians valuable time. Review key aspects of the patient's history with the patient, so he or she feels comfortable that you know his or her history. This will increase a patient's confidence. Inquire about current medications and their effects. In short, show that the person is not just a number;

- **Show concern**. You can achieve the perception of caring in three simple steps: having eye contact, listening attentively, and calling the patient by name;

- **Present options**. Patients value honest and full disclosure. Give the facts and present various options. Allow the patient to be a partner in making treatment decisions, or at least explain why you are taking a certain course and what options you have eliminated;

- **Put it in writing**. During exams, many patients are a bundle of nerves. They may forget almost everything you have said, so write down important treatment plans; and

- **Bring closure**. Let the patient — not you — end the exam. Before you leave, answer questions, listen and ask, "Have you received what you needed today?"

Timely follow-up

When physicians order tests, patients want to hear the results as soon as possible. If the patient is ill, had a procedure, or is anxious, a courtesy call to see how the patient is doing will build confidence in the physician and the system.

- **Notification of test results**: You should send normal test results in writing by the time promised. If the results are abnormal, call immediately. Explain the results and any required follow-up. Patients worry. They will call many times if you do not take control of the process and arrange for a time to get results back to patients; and

- **Courtesy telephone calls**: Make it a practice to identify key patients each day to call the following day. Usually one or two patients will stand out each day as key. It may be because they had a procedure or because they were extremely anxious. The criteria each physician uses to identify key patients is not as important as remembering to have nurse call one or two key patients each day to see how they are doing. Patients truly appreciate these calls.

Appropriate and timely billing

Bills should be understandable and clear. It should not take an MBA to figure how much a patient owes, or an MPH to understand what services were provided. The bill should state whether a person on staff will contact the insurance company or whether you expect the patient to handle the insurance. Patients also expect clear communication about when the bill is due, what forms of payment you accept, who can answer questions or discuss concerns, and who they should call if they have questions.

Having a clear vision for the future and understanding the needs of your patients prepares you for the next step of developing systems to support the patient encounter.

The following chapters will guide you through a process of developing essential systems a successful medical practice needs. It is important that management, physicians and staff work together to develop practical systems that support efficient, effective patient care. It also is important that patients perceive value from each interaction with your organization.

Read on with an open mind. Think about how you can use the six guiding principles to improve the value of care at your health care organization.

◆

Chapter 6

Making a time commitment

◆

Determining the amount of time each physician will spend at work seeing clinic patients is the first step in making a time commitment to the practice. Making this commitment is the conscious, deliberate act of deciding how many hours each physician plans to be available, day-by-day, week-by-week and year-by-year to see patients.

Time, after all, is the "product" that physicians have to sell in their practice. How much of their life they choose to spend in their practice is up to each physician. However, it is vitally important to make a commitment in specific, measurable terms.

Committing a set number of hours to each physician's practice does not guarantee that patients will fill each open slot. It does, however, give you a measurable target, a place to start and an important benchmark for practice measurement.

Taking a time inventory also will help management calculate the level of resources needed to support each practice. Volume of work directly relates to the time each physician allocates to seeing patients. Low productivity often relates to excess time away from the office.

Over the last 10 years, we have noted that several physicians with dwindling practices simply spent too much time away from the office. If you carefully document each physician's time away from the office, you will know exactly the number of days per year each physician should spend in the clinic seeing patients.

How do you calculate the time each physician will spend in the office? Simply start with the number of days in a year, then reduce that number by taking out weekends, vacations, holidays and professional development seminars.

It is amazing how fast 365 days dwindle. Here is an example:

Available clinic days (sample worksheet)	
365	Total days per year
-104	Weekend days
-6	Holidays
-20	Vacation days
-20	Professional days
215	Available days

Now that you know each physician will work 215 days per year in the clinic seeing patients, you can determine how may patients per day each physician must see to meet his or her goal.

Let's assume the goal is 4,500 office visits per year per physician and each physician plans to see those patents in 215 days. That equals 21 patients per day per physician. If each physician averages two "no-shows" per day and if you add those two to the 21 patients actually seen each day, each physician's goal per day would be 23 scheduled patient-care visits. The following worksheet helps calculate the number of scheduled patient-care visits needed per day.

Office visit goals (sample worksheet)	
4,500	Total annual office visits
divided by 215	Available days
equals 21	Average patients per day
plus 2	Average "no-shows" per day
equals 23	Average scheduled office visits per day
times 20 minutes per patient	Average minute per visit
equals 460 minutes per day	Average minutes
divided by 60 equal 7.7 hours of time that needs to be scheduled per day	Available hours per day

As you can see from the above example, we continued the process of identifying the available hours of scheduled time per day to accomplish the goal. To complete the above work worksheet, you must first identify the average length of time physicians spend with each patient.

Continuous Stop Watch Time Study

Several different methodologies can be used to determine this number. In our studies we use the Continuous Stop Watch Time Study methodology. An outside observer actually watching and recording the time the physician spends with each patient is the unique characteristic of this methodology. This methodology is more accurate and gives you the opportunity to identify all the components of a patient visit, not just the face-to-face time. For our studies, we include the following in a patient visit:

- reviewing the chart;

- spending face-to-face time with the patient;

- dictating;

- completing the chart and charge ticket;

- talking with family members; and

- reviewing test results.

A sample of the tool we use is on the following page.

A continuous study means you start the stop watch as the physician begins in the morning and stop it once he or she finishes in the evening. Each time the physician changes tasks you record the task and when he or she completes that task you record the time.

When the study is complete, subtract the time from the time above to get the task time. Summarize all task times on a summary sheet and record the total number of patients seen. If you divide the number of patients into the total of the six tasks that make up a complete patient visit, you will arrive at the average number of minutes per patient visit. A copy of the Observation Summary sheet is on page 33 so you can see how this is done.

Continuous Stop Watch Time Study

Physician: John Doe, M.D.
Scheduled patients: 21
Add-ons: 4
No-shows/cancels: 3

Department: FP
Date: 2/17/94
Total patients seen: 22

Description	Reading	Normal time	Task code	Skill level	Comments
1 Personal time	13.50	13.50	Pt	—	Late
2 Misc. paperwork	15.04	1.54	11	RN	
3 In with #1 patient	25.03	9.99	2	MD	
4 Misc. paperwork	25.43	.40	11	OA	
5 Chart #1	26.14	.71	4	MD	
6 Communicate with MD	28.72	2.58	7	MD	
7 Communicate with OA	31.69	2.97	9	MD	
8 In with #2 patient	44.57	12.88	2	MD	
9 **Totals**					

Observation Summary Sheet

Physician: John Doe, MD
Date: 2/17/94

Clinic patients: 10
Add-on: 4
Cancel/no show: 3
Hospital patients: 7

01 - review chart
02 - with patient
03 - dictate
04 - complete chart/chg. ticket
05 - communicate with family
06 - review tests

07 - communicate with MD
08 - comm. with patient/family (not seen)
09 - communicate with staff
10 - communicate with outside organization
11 - misc. paperwork
12 - non-MD task

13 - looking for something
AI - analyst interrupt
IT - idle time
PT - personal time
L - lunch

Title	01	02	03	04	05	06	07	08	09	10	11	12	13	AI	It	PT	L
Time in	0.29	9.99		0.71		4.11	2.97				0.40		0.87	1.54	4.44	13.50	82.35
Minutes		12.88		1.91			0.25				0.99		0.30	2.58		1.48	
		9.15		1.51			0.68				3.07		0.44	1.28		1.63	
		13.96		1.79			0.97							19.52			
		22.05		2.85										1.15			
		15.26		1.92										15.69			
		13.82		1.47										2.87			
		4.42		1.16										3.14			
		14.60		1.17										1.44			
		9.93		1.85													
		10.24		1.11													
	0.29	136.60	0.00	17.45	0.00	4.11	4.87	0.00	0.00	0.00	4.46	0.00	1.61	49.21	4.44	16.61	82.35
Freq.		10															
Time/PT		13.66															

Total # PT seen	10	
PT time	158.5	(1-6)
PT hours	2.64	/60
Ave/min/PT	15.85	

Total non/productive	154.22	(12-L)
Total productive	167.78	(1-11)
Productive hours	2.8	/60
Total time study time	322.00 Minutes	5.4 Hours

Codes 01 - 06 make up complete patient visit

Self-analysis tool

A second method for acquiring the information is a self-analysis tool. While this method is not as accurate as the stop watch method, physicians can complete this task independently. Attach the following form to each chart and monitor for several weeks. Begin recording times when the patient goes into the exam room. Note the time each person interacts with the patient and record the time under the "in" column. Also record the time each person leaves the room under the "out" column. Subtract the "out" column from the "in" column to arrive at your task time. Do the same procedure for the other tasks.

Self-analysis tool			
Task	In	Out	Task time
Patient			
Nurse			
Physician			
Dictation/ charting/ charge ticket			
Review test results			

If the average time each physician spends with each patient visit is 20 minutes, each physician will need 460 minutes or 7.7 hours of available patient-care time per day as shown in the original work sheet.

Remember to monitor the number of days physicians actually work in the clinic seeing patients and the number of patients seen each day. Working fewer days than the stated number of days per year and/or seeing fewer patients per day than the goal is the major reason for decreased annual revenue. In a capitated system the result of physicians seeing fewer patients than their goal will result in the need to add more physicians. This could jeopardize the income of the remaining physicians.

Basic as this groundwork sounds, many physicians do not know how many days they have worked in the clinic the past year, let alone how many patients they have seen. When physicians guess at the number of patients they see per week, the number is invariably high. Physicians tend to think back to their busiest days, then project that same volume to the rest of the schedule.

In declining practices, failure to monitor patient volumes and days worked are common problems. Having a goal for a set number of patients per day benefits the physician in both a fee-for-service and managed care environment. There is simply no better yardstick for measuring productivity.

In a fee-for-service environment, time inventories allow you to:

- forecast revenue by estimating dollars-per-visit times visits-per-year;

- share tangible productivity goals with staff and motivate those who keep the schedule full; and

- allocate staff to volume.

In a managed care environment, time inventories help to:

- build realistic targets for patient panel size, based on frequency and length of appointments;

- forecast potential revenue by knowing how large a panel size for which you can contract; and

- monitor the utilization of the patient panel and provide reports to insurance companies or firms contracting for care.

It is imperative not only to identify the number of hours each physician will spend in the clinic each week, but also monitor his or her accessibility. If patients call and the support staff tells them they cannot be seen for months, something is wrong.

Support staff should identify at the end of each week exactly how soon each physician can see non-urgent patients. Remember our guidelines from Chapter Three? We often see practices that have time to see patients; however, there are so many barriers in their schedules, that it is not easy to fit patients into their schedules.

Sometimes physicians can see more patients but the limitation in their practice is the amount of work the support staff can handle. It may be caused by having too few support staff, but more often it is the result of having a practice that is out of balance. This is not acceptable. You should never limit a practice by the amount of work your support staff members can handle.

Another common limitation we see is the support staff members protecting a physician by limiting the number of patients seen in one day. Staff members often protect the schedule out of concern for the physician or themselves. Unfortunately we have seen times when the support staff have literally protected the physician out of business.

It is very dangerous, especially in today's environment, ever to close a practice to new patients. Practices limit themselves. When access reaches a level that is not acceptable to a patient, they will seek care somewhere else. In a capitated managed care environment where each physician has a clearly defined patient panel, closing a practice is acceptable. However, few physicians have an accurate picture of the true number of patients in their practice at any given time. Patients leave for various reasons, oftentimes the physician and staff are never aware of the change.

Physicians who have closed their practices to new patients for as little as six months, often have a difficult time rebuilding the practice.

Take a time inventory by using the sample forms on the following pages. By making a time commitment in specific, measurable terms, you will have taken the first important step in building a successful practice.

Available clinic days **(worksheet)**	
365	Total days per year
	Weekend days
	Holidays
	Vacation days
	Professional days
	Available days
	Personal time

Office visit goals **(worksheet)**	
	Total annual office visits
	Available days
	Average patients per day
	Average no-shows per day
	Average scheduled office visits per day
	Average minutes per visit
	Available minutes per day
	Available hours per day

Continuous Stop Watch Time Study

Physician:
Scheduled patients:
Add-ons:
No-shows/cancels:

Department:
Date:
Total patients seen:

Description	Reading	Normal time	Task code	Skill level	Comments
1					
2					
3					
4					
5					
6					
7					
8					
9					
10					
11					
12					
13					
14					
15					
Totals					

Observation summary

Physician:
Date:

Clinic patients:
Add-on:
Cancel/no show:
Hospital patients:

01 - review chart
02 - with patient
03 - dictate
04 - complete chart/chg. ticket
05 - communicate with family
06 - review tests

07 - communicate with MD
08 - comm. with patient/family (not seen)
09 - communicate with staff
10 - communicate with outside organization
11 - Misc. paperwork
12 - non-MD task

13 - looking for something
AI - analyst interrupt
IT - idle time
PT - personal time
L - lunch

Title	01	02	03	04	05	06	07	08	09	10	11	12	13	AI	IT	PT	L
Time in																	
Minutes																	
	0.00	0.00	0.00	0.00	0.00	0.00	0.00	0.00	0.00	0.00	0.00	0.00	0.00	0.00	0.00	0.00	0.00
Freq.																	
Time/PT																	

Total # PT seen			
PT time	0.0	(1-6)	
PT hours	0.0	/60	

Total non/PR		(12-L)
Total prod	0.0	(1-11)
Prod hrs	0.0	/60
Total time study time	0.00 Minutes	(1-L)

Ave/min/PT   0.00 Minutes

Codes 01 - 06 make up complete patient visit

Chapter 7

Balancing work loads

Balanced work load is a key ingredient of a successful practice.

Having about the same number of physicians available on any given day results in predictable work loads in a practice. This leads to a steady, measured use of support staff and helps set the framework of a steady flow of patients through the practice from day to day.

If this kind of balance seems like too abstract a concept, consider a simple analogy: driving in a car.

When all four tires have the same amount of pressure the car is in balance. It runs smoothly. When one tire is flat, the car erratically careens down the road. It pulls to one side, even though the other tires have perfect tread and the exact recommended tire pressure.

For the car to run smoothly, it needs the balance of all four tires hitting the road at the same time with the same pressure.

The same is true of a medical practice: balance can make the difference between a place that runs smoothly, or a place that is chaotic.

It is easy to overlook this uneven physician staffing level in diagnosing a dysfunctional practice — but often it is a contributing factor.

What difference does it make if you have the same number of physicians available whenever the practice is open?

Staffing the same number of physicians from day to day evenly distributes work loads throughout the week. In practices without balanced physician coverage, wildly varying day-to-day fluctuations in capacity can occur. This means that staff are either overwhelmed with more patients than they can handle, or bored with non-productive idle time.

This uncertainty — the feast or famine in the flow of patients — turns work into a roller coaster for the staff. It's no wonder the staff at such practices are edgy, uptight and often curt with patients.

The patient ultimately bears the brunt of this lack of planning and forethought. The patient is either rushed through the system, left unattended in the exam room or ignored for too long in the waiting room.

When a patient experiences this rude treatment from clinic staff members, he or she may not say anything immediately, but just wait.

Some studies show that when a person experiences poor service, he or she will tell 27 other people about it. This is word-of-mouth advertising gone amok.

The patient will talk about it. "The long wait" will be the topic of many a dinner conversation, a party tidbit, and an item on the agenda when a friend asks for a physician referral.

"I can tell you where not to go," will be the answer.

Fundamentally, uneven staffing increases the chances of providing inconsistent or poor service to patients, who are the very reasons a practice exists.

In smaller practices, balanced staffing occurs informally. "Oh, you are taking your vacation then. Well, I will schedule mine a few weeks after you get back."

In medium-sized practices where communication among providers is not as personal or frequent, problems start to occur. Often in large multispecialty clinics, no single person knows what the roster of physicians in is on any given day.

The solution: select a central person to manage a clinic-wide master schedule to track staffing every single day of the year. You should structure the schedule to guarantee even coverage while accommodating physicians' vacations, professional development, research and other activities.

However, remember that patients' needs come first.

The staffing must be adequate to sustain a balanced flow of patients through the practice.

Take a moment and see how this works in practice. The graph on page 45 shows a practice where day-to-day variations range from 84 to 178 patient visits. This particular clinic staffed the same each day.

What should the accurate staffing volume be?

The mathematical average is 120 patients per day. If that actually held true, about one-third of the time the practice would be short-staffed.

If one person checks in all your patients and your volume rises from 84 to 176 patient visits, there will be a lineup in the waiting area. On the days when the volume drops, there are wasted labor hours.

Who suffers the most on the days that you are either over- or understaffed?

In the short run, the patient suffers.

However, it will not be long until the entire practice suffers. Word will get out that this practice does not provide good service.

Balance in staffing makes good business sense. It avoids staff turnover and assures astute use of labor. It is good for physicians because they can operate in a more predictable environment without feeling rushed. Most importantly, keeping a balanced master schedule results in good service to patients.

The following graph shows one example of the day-to-day variability in staffing. A copy of a balanced master schedule also follows.

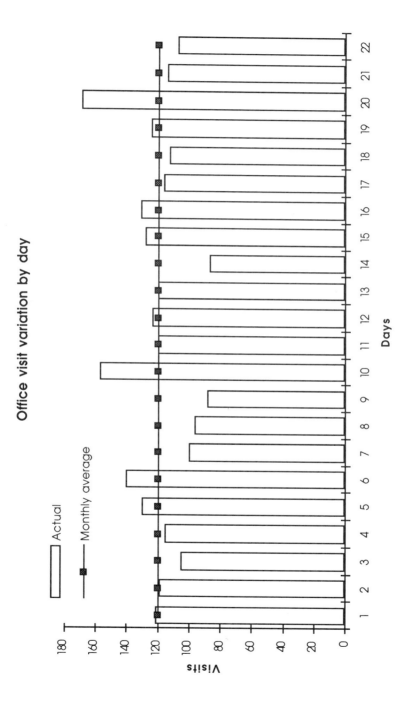

Office visit variation by day

Master schedule

Provider	Mon. am	Mon. pm	Tues. am	Tues. pm	Wed. am	Wed. pm	Thurs. am	Thurs. pm	Fri. am	Fri. pm
MD1	South	South	South	S(QOW)/off	South	South	South	South	South	South
MD2	Main	Main	West	West	Main	Main	Main	Main	Main	Main
MD3	S	S	Main	Main	Main	Main	Main	Main	Main	Main
MD4	Main	Main	Main	Main	Main	Main	Main	Main	S	S
MD5	Main	Main	Main	Main	S	Main	Main	Off	Main	Main
MD6	Main	Main	Main	Main	Main	S	Main	Main	Main	Main
MD7	Main	Main	S	South	Main	Main	Off	Main	Main	Main
MD8	East	East	Off	S(QOW)/off	East	East	West	West	East	East
MD9	West	West	Main	Main	West	West	S	S	West	West
AHP	South	South	South	South	South	South	South	South	South	South
AHP	Main	Main	East	East	Off	Off	East	East	Main	Main
AHP	Main	Main	Main	Main	Off	Main	Main	Main	Off	Off
AHP	West	West	West	West	West	West	West	West	West	West
AHP	Off	Off	Main	Main	Main	Main	Main	Main	Main	Main
Main	7	7	7	7	7	7	7	7	7	7
East	1	1	1	1	1	1	1	1	1	1
South	2	2	2	2	2	2	2	2	2	2
West	2	2	2	2	2	2	2	2	2	2
Surgery	1	1	1	1	1	1	1	1	1	1

Code:
S = Surgery

◆

Chapter 8

Decreasing unnecessary variation

◆

It is important that you lay the groundwork for a smooth practice by decreasing unnecessary variation within your organization. Physicians tend to develop very different systems because we ask them *how* they want things done rather than what their *needs and expectations* are for different systems. Most physicians tell me they really do not care how things are done as long as they get the job done. They also say that the only reason they do it the way they do is because someone asked them how they wanted it done. Rarely do we develop systems based on the needs of our physicians. We let the physicians tell us how they want things done.

Long before scheduling the first appointment, you should implement systems that will make the best use of the physician's time. (Of course, in existing practices, it is never too late to put new systems in place.) Ask your physicians what their needs are from various systems.

Some of the most important systems include the following steps.

Establish an appropriate appointment-scheduling system

Many physicians have built successful appointment scheduling systems by implementing this formula. This recipe-like approach may seem simple, but it has worked time and again. Here is how it works:

First, call a brainstorming meeting of all the physicians who will be practicing together and using the same support staff. In a large group practice, this might be a specialty or a section.

The purpose of this meeting is to categorize appointments by length of time it takes for the physician to see the patient. Our time studies show that the length of time a physician spends with his or her patients that come in for the same reason is very consistent.

Try to list the reason for visits from most frequent to least frequent. It is important to be specific and thorough, but far more important that the higher volume visits are accurate, since a majority of the physician's time is spent with those patients. However, do not forget those infrequent events, especially if they take a lot of the physician's time.

Next put each of these visits into one of three categories: short, medium or long. Sometimes physicians find they need four or five categories. Even if some physicians only want to see all their visits in two categories (for example, 15 minutes and 30 minutes). Still, break it down into the maximum number of categories any physician needs. The time physicians choose to see patients can be different for each physician. However, the consistency comes with the type of patients seen in each category. This way training for support staff is consistent. For instance, if a person was coming in for a physical with no problems, schedule it under the same category for all physicians. The following shows how you can have the same categories of appointments and yet each physician can assign the length of time that is appropriate for their style.

Type of visit				
Brief (BV)	Intermediate (IV)	Extended (EV)	Comprehensive (CV)	Complex (CX)
MD1 10	20	30	40	50
MD2 10	10	20	20	30
in minutes				

There may be discussions about whether you can provide a particular service in a short, medium or long visit. While some compromise is necessary, natural groupings of visits by the amount of time they take to provide typically emerge. Only use physician's time. Often we see appointment times built with support time included. Again this is an example of letting your support staff time dictate the volume of patients you can see.

Next decide what is unique about each of these categories. Some groups feel new patients are unique because you must develop a new data base and it takes more time. Consultations are usually unique because you not only need to build a new data base, but you also must review outside records. Begin to build criteria for patients that fall under each category. On the following page you can see a partial set of categories that one of our groups chose.

Notice the remarks column in our example. Place standardized key information in this field. This is the information the back office support staff will need when preparing the chart and room for the patient visit. Remember, the proactive approach saves physician time.

Appointment types and criteria

Abbreviation	Appointment name	Description	Remarks
New	New patient visit	New data base evaluation	Date of last physical
Con	Consult	Referred from another provider or seeking a second opinion	Referring provider/have outside records been ordered/date of last exam/problem
BV	Brief visit	Simple problem (see below) or follow-up of recent visit	Primary care provider/ chief complaint/duration
EV	Extended visit	Multiple problems or new patients that do not want a complete evaluation or return data base evaluation or any problem not listed under BV	Date of last exam/list problems or state no problems

Conditions appropriate for brief visit (BV) include the following:
Rash
Conjunctivitis
Ear ache
Sore throat
Cough
Wound check
Post op

Next comes the step that allows physicians to have control over their practices and determine their own practice styles. Each physician can assign the length of time he or she needs for each of these categories. The time must match their practice style.

For example, a physician who tends to work very quietly and swiftly may allow 10 minutes for short appointments, while another provider who likes to spend more time may allocate 15 minutes for short visits. However, if the physician only spends 10 minutes and uses a 15 minute interval for patients, he or she is losing 5 minutes per patient each day. This will make a tremendous difference in the number of patients a physician can care for in a year.

By using the information from the Continuous Stop Watch Time Study that we discussed in Chapter Six, "Making a time commitment," you can use those times to help determine the category times. The time study will help measure the actual amounts of time physicians spend on various procedures and with various appointments. You can determine the time a physician needs from this study.

If you build appropriate appointment types, you can develop logical thought processes to help the staff schedule more effectively. This process is known as a rules-based approach to appointment scheduling.

Consider the benefits of going through this exercise. It helps the telephone staff move logically from a caller's need to reason for visit, to criteria for visit and then to book an appropriate amount of time for any type of appointment. Rules-based approach allows flexibility for physicians to write rules that help direct questions to the patient so that the answer to some key questions automatically places a patient in a particular appointment type. This allows for accurate centralized scheduling and restores physicians' confidence in the schedulers.

By starting from the patient's point of view — the reason for calling — you can build in triaging that helps your staff ask meaningful questions and schedule patients for the appropriate amounts of time.

In building schedules, many physicians set aside time each day just before lunch or at the end of the day for urgent-care cases. Building in this time allows a practice to respond quickly if urgent care is needed. If these slots do not fill, the physician can finish up paper work or take a longer lunch. These are the least predictable appointments. Therefore, when you add patients earlier in the day, it forces all patients scheduled after the addition to wait. This inconveniences many patients.

One word of caution: some practices try to restrict their schedules. For example, a physician might allow a "new-patient" slot at 9 a.m. only. This creates a barrier to new patient access. In general, these arbitrary appointment requirements clog the system, cause otherwise revenue-producing schedule slots to go unfilled and frustrate patients.

We recommend open schedules that do not assign types of patients to certain times a day. Experience shows that an open, patient-focused scheduling system is better than building a restricted one, as long as you match the appointment time to the physicians' style. In this way, you accept any patient any time, regardless of the reason, as long as the amount of time available matches the anticipated length of services.

Many physicians feel it is not possible to make the determination. Try the system — it works.

The very act of developing this appointment system is a team-building exercise and the result — a well-designed appointment scheduling system — will reap rewards in efficiency for years to come. Most scheduling systems result in long patient waits, both for an appointment and for the exam. This one will not.

Developing an effective scheduling system will enhance both physicians' and support staffs' productivity.

Prepare for appointments in a systematic way

Several days prior to the appointment, your support staff should begin to pull charts. The day before the visit support staff should review the medical records of the patient scheduled the next day to assure completeness and accuracy. If the patient is coming from another facility, make sure outside records arrive before the day of the appointment. Everything should be up to date. The physician should never have to come out of an exam room to retrieve missing information from a medical record.

Keep all exam rooms well stocked

Stock each exam room appropriately so that each physician can complete an entire visit without leaving the room to retrieve items. Stock all exam rooms identically, including the placement and organization of patient-education materials. That way, a physician does not spend time fumbling through cabinets. Physicians should agree on what supplies, equipment and educational materials to place in all rooms. This uniformity saves money, keeps supplies current, simplifies exam room stocking and allows physicians the flexibility of using any room in the area.

Stock every exam room at least daily.

Develop protocols for rooming patients

Develop protocols for greeting patients, taking vital signs, gathering other important information (such as allergies) and writing down the presenting complaint.

Protocols should answer questions, such as "Does this patient need to:

- have blood pressure taken?"

- be weighed?"

- be dressed in a gown?" or

- complete any forms prior to the physician's visit?"

Clearly, each staff member will bring his or her own personality to this task, but it is vital to emphasize that this initial contact with the patient establishes the tone of the visit.

Treat patients with respect, call them by name and make them feel as if you hear and care about their complaints. Give the patient information on why requests are being made and help them understand what to expect when they see the physician. Help the patients focus on the true reason for needing to see the physician. Patients often are very vague and waste a great deal of the physician's time getting to the real problem.

This proactive, courteous, professional yet friendly approach to rooming a patient is a key factor in patient satisfaction and improved physician efficiency.

A sample form is on page 57.

Outline the steps
for discharging patients

(Discharging is the word we use for dealing with orders and follow-up after the physician sees the patient).

Equally important to rooming a patient is a smooth, friendly and efficient discharge. A written order sheet will activate the discharge. You can find a sample order sheet in Chapter 10, "Creating a team — interdependency." The order sheet includes various tests that might be ordered, educational materials needed, required referrals and follow-up needs.

Whatever the next step, write it on the order sheet. This is infinitely more effective than calling out orders to staff who must scramble to jot down information.

The order sheet becomes the test verification form. Once the support staff members execute the orders, immediately place the order sheet in a tickler file for test verification and follow-up. Test verification is the act of checking to see that all tests ordered were completed and results returned to the office. When test results return, check them off the order sheet and you have completed the test verification task.

The order sheet also should tell the support staff how to notify the patient of the results. Physicians usually want to review all test results when they come back. However, if the order sheet is used appropriately, the physician does not have to get involved with the process if the tests are normal.

While conducting the exam, the physician can write instructions and talk with the patient at the same time. For example, the physician might say, "I am recommending that you see Dr. Back, a specialist in the treatment of spine disease," as he jots it down on the order sheet.

Rooming criteria

Category	Reason for visit	HT	WT	VS	LMP	Meds	T	Expose area of concern	Undress completely	UA	Outside records
New	PE	X	X	X	X	X			X	X	
CONS		X	X	X	X	X			X		X
BV	Follow-up										
	Pain			X		X	X	X			
	Cough		X	X		X	X	X			
	Diarrhea			X		X	X	X			
EV	RPE	X	X	X	X	X	X	X	X	X	
	New problem		X	X	X	X					

This is an incomplete sample. Build criteria based on your patient base.

As the appointment concludes, the physician can give the form to the patient to give to the support staff, who knows instantly what actions the instructions should trigger. Patients appreciate a copy of this form to help them comply with the orders.

Make a practice of prompt documentation after each patient

After each patient visit, the physician should promptly complete these tasks:

- Finish any dictation (recording the information is five-times faster than writing it out);

- Complete the charge ticket and any necessary billing documentation;

- Check the message clipboard for any ASAP messages (details on message handling follow under "Win the battle over paperwork"); and

- Review the chart for the next appointment.

In the midst of the patient care, there are two important, ongoing functions that play an important role in any efficient practice: paper work and handling the telephones.

Both deserve a plan.

Win the battle over paper work

Delayed paperwork causes rework. Time is sapped from a practice when physicians must make multiple copies of an order, request or notice; or when staff members must field several telephone calls from a patient for one prescription that is buried in the bottom of an "in" box.

One solution is to educate support staff members to use a low-tech but effective system that assigns a priority to every piece of information before channeling it to physicians. This process keeps information moving smoothly throughout the day, from staff to physician and back to staff, without interrupting the physician or causing pileups.

With so much information flowing through a practice, a priority system is essential.

An efficient system is as easy as providing every support staff member and physician with sheets of adhesive colored dots and three mailboxes, labeled "in," "out" and "action." Also place "ASAP" clipboards, or just clips, between the exam rooms.

Staff members triage information for physicians, sorting all paper, requests and messages into a hierarchy of priorities. To minimize interruptions, staff should put questions in writing.

Here are the uses for each of the three boxes and the ASAP clip.

Use ASAP clips for items that need an action completed between patients or for quick signatures. The rule is if it only takes 10 seconds to act on the message, put it on the ASAP clip. This will facilitate paper flow throughout the day. A good example is the prescription refill that only needs a quick signature, yet often ends up at the bottom of an "in" box. The delay in responding to the message triggers several additional telephone calls. To help maintain good customer service, place patient information requests that may not be urgent but are easy to answer quickly in the ASAP clip.

Action box is for all items that need resolution before the end of the day.

The "in" box is for all other paper work that the physician needs or requests to see. Encourage your physicians to empty all "in" boxes each Friday to avoid a monumental task in the future. Many physicians spend Saturday cleaning out their "in" boxes. It is amazing what you will find.

The "out" box should be emptied hourly by support staff. As physicians act on ASAP and action items during the course of the day, they place them in their "out" box. As part of the work flow, whomever rooms patients also empties "out" boxes.

Even though this seems basic, emptying "out" boxes is one of the hardest things for staff members to remember.

Marked with color-coded dots, these papers and messages take the support staff a matter of seconds to dispatch. They include items needing only a signature, changes of schedule or urgent notes. (The registered nurse should determine the urgency of a message.)

Put first things first

To further reduce inefficiency, support staff should direct telephone and mail traffic.

Opening mail

From a productivity perspective, support staff should open the mail and respond to as much as they can, giving the physicians only what they need.

Phone triage

Train staff to determine priorities. Managers should write criteria for what should go into action boxes. Phone messages rarely go into the in box. The receptionist usually routes emergency and urgent calls to a registered nurse who can determine their level of urgency. Registered nurses can handle most telephone calls, freeing up time for the physician to see more patients.

Phone messages

Phone message forms can help signal immediately what kind of action is required. Clinics should use different kinds of forms for telephone messages: one form for prescriptions, one for personal calls and one for patient encounters, with a duplicate that goes into a patient record.

Put it in writing

Encourage staff to put things in writing and avoid interrupting physicians. Interruptions cause delays. Remember to always develop systems that support efficiency and make the best use of a physician's time.

Follow-up is mandatory

Repeatedly, physicians say that they have a deep-seated fear that something may fall through the cracks — a test result may not get communicated, a prescription may not be ordered as promised, documentation may be misplaced. This can lead to disgruntled patients and in some cases, can even put the practice in jeopardy of a lawsuit.

Precise, documented, well-maintained systems not only make things flow more smoothly, but also guarantee that tasks are routinely completed.

To prepare systems that streamline physicians' time, put in place these elements.

A good patient-flow system should include:

- greeting;

- visit prep;

- room stocking;

- rooming criteria;

- order execution; and

- follow-up.

Communication systems should include:

- "in," "out" and "action" boxes for the physician along with ASAP clips between exam rooms;

- message identification, prioritization and flow system;

- tickler systems for patient communication, including reporting test results, scheduling appointments and sending reminders of services needed;

- tracking services and charges so billing can occur in a timely, accurate manner; and

- telephone protocols, including the use of a registered nurse to triage patient calls.

Housekeeping, storage and stocking for efficiency include:

- keeping adequate supplies on hand; and

- keeping all exam rooms well-stocked, with supplies in uniform places from room to room.

Create a special meetings calendar

Keep a master calendar of all mandatory meetings, days working in other locations and any other non-daily activity that periodically occurs in the physician's schedule. This is very helpful to keep from forgetting to add a meeting to the schedule and inadvertently scheduling patients. When this happens, it not only frustrates physicians, it inconveniences the patient that has to be rescheduled. It also creates a great deal of rework which is very costly to an organization.

One last comment about rescheduling patients — they hate it and may use it as a reason to find another physician. Planning ahead and setting up effective systems will help to alleviate the need to reschedule patients.

◆

Chapter 9

Distributing tasks appropriately

◆

Develop a "job description" for the health care practitioners and support staff

To work at optimal efficiency, a practice needs appropriate people, doing appropriate tasks, within the appropriate time frames.

An easy way to identify current tasks is by using the Statement of Duties tool on the following page.

This tool provides an organized format for obtaining employees' and practitioners' impressions of what tasks they are doing in their present position. Each employee and practitioner should complete this form in the following way:

- Enter employee's or practitioner's name, job title, department name and date;

- Identify the key process — the purpose for hiring the person. The key process differs from the job title in that it explains what process the employee is actually doing. One example may be the receptionist. You hire a receptionist to check in patients, yet the job title is receptionist;

- Identify the key volume indicator. This is what drives the volume of work. Using the receptionist as an example again, the number of patient appointments drives the volume of work for the receptionist;

- Have each employee and practitioner list all tasks they perform, whether they do the task on a daily, weekly, monthly or yearly basis;

- Estimate the number of times the employee completes the task on a weekly basis;

Statement of Duties

Name: Jane Doe

Title: receptionist

Key process: prepare
charts and check in patients
Date: 2/94

Department:
Family practice
Key volume indicator:
Patients seen

Task	Volume per week	How counted	Skill level
Check in charts	500	Each chart	Clerical — low
Prepare charts	500	Each chart	Clerical — low
Check in patients	480	Patients seen	Receptionist

- Document the method for counting each task. For example, the receptionist checks in patients — count each patient checked in for an appointment; and

- Determine the most appropriate skill level to perform the task. It is important to identify each job classification's scope of practice, to assure appropriate use of different types of employees. This will vary from state to state.

The Statement of Duties form is a key tool when analyzing a practice. It is helpful to use a patient's visit through the office as a tool for categorizing the tasks associated with an appointment. The categories include triaging, scheduling, obtaining medical records, admitting, rooming, diagnosing and treating, teaching, discharging, following up and billing.

So how do you go about creating job descriptions?

Within each of the tasks required as a patient moves through the system, list everything that needs to happen to make that part of the visit go smoothly. Determine who on the team — clerk, medical assistant, registered nurse — has the appropriate skill level to carry out the task.

Once each employee completes his or her form, you should know all the work associated with each patient as well as tasks that are being done that do not relate to the patient visit. You also will have a list of the appropriate skill level for each task. With this information you can determine the most appropriate employee to perform each task. The last step is to develop job descriptions.

To identify the actual number of employees you need in each job, time study each task. The more repetitive and consistent the task, the less number of samples you need to feel the time is valid and reliable. If the task times vary considerably, you will need a larger sample of times.

By using the identified task time multiplied by an estimate of how many appointments you anticipate each day, you can determine how much time each of these tasks will take and how many employees of each skill level you will need in your practice.

Finally, besides the tasks that are driven by the number of patients you see, there also is ongoing work that needs to be done, regardless of your patient volume. These fixed tasks include things such as opening and sorting mail, stocking exam rooms and providing reception and phone coverage.

Identify the time per day to perform each task and allocate an average time per day for these tasks. You can identify the number of employees you need to staff both the phones and the reception desk by determining the volume of work per day. Remember, you must minimally staff these positions based on the hours of operation. The following example emphasizes the need to look beyond the task time.

Suppose the time study shows you only need five hours of receptionist time to do the tasks you have assigned that job, however, the clinic is open eight hours per day. You must staff the reception desk eight hours each day and try to bring other tasks to the receptionist that she or he can do when not checking in patients.

By defining the roles, responsibilities and appropriate skill levels required for each staff person's job, you have taken another step towards building an effective medical practice.

Look at the physician's time

What should a physician do? How should he or she spend time in the office? Or, perhaps more importantly, what shouldn't a physician be doing? Our research shows that in the most productive and profitable practices, a physician confines the majority of his or her time to these key tasks:

- reviewing patients' medical records;

- conducting medical exams and performing procedures;

- developing and communicating treatment plans;

- documenting information, treatment plans and services;

- communicating with the patients' families or significant others;

- reviewing tests results; and

- coding charge tickets.

Physicians who routinely spend time on other tasks may be wasting time unwittingly.

The litmus test of an activity that justifies a physician's time is this: "Is this a task that someone else could safely, legally and effectively complete?" If the answer is yes, then the physician should not be routinely doing that task.

What should a registered nurse do?

A registered nurse is a great asset to any practice if used appropriately and a great expense if used inappropriately. Appropriate telephone triage will save a practice valuable time and money. While other health care workers often call patients back after talking with the physician, registered nurses have the ability to handle telephone triage independently. Constant interruptions dramatically slow down a practice. Allowing a nurse to handle daily phone calls increases physician's productivity.

Our research shows that in many cases the registered nurse can save a physician up to two hours a day just by handling all the patient problem telephone calls. This will allow the physician more time to see patients in the office.

Patient education is another task for the registered nurse. While education is extremely important, it also is very time consuming. Allowing your registered nurse to do the patient education will also free up the physician to see more patients in the office.

You also can delegate to your registered nurse such tasks as minor procedures and patient assessments.

Remember, clerical support staff should complete most of the clerical work.

Distributing tasks appropriately and delegating tasks to the lowest skill level person that can perform the task safely and legally is a good business move. However, even more importantly, it will improve morale. When employees and physicians are working at their potential, they are able to focus on better patient care.

Statement of Duties

Name:
Title:
Key process:
Date:

Department:
Key volume indicator:

Task	Volume per week	How counted	Skill level

◆

Chapter 10

Creating a team — interdependency

◆

Teamwork
Coming together is a beginning;
Keeping together is progress;
Working together is success.
— Henry Ford

The key to any well-functioning medical practice is teamwork. Patients expect the same quality of care each time they come to the office. It makes sense to develop systems that allow for continuity of care when either the physician or his/her support staff are out of the office.

However, when we bring this up to physicians, they usually say, "My patients only want to talk to my nurse."

Because we heard this comment so often, we decided to ask patients if this was true. For the most part they preferred to talk with their physician's nurse if they could not talk to their doctor. Upon further questioning, they invariably stated that what was most important to them was talking with someone who could answer their questions without having to be put on hold or transferred to someone else. When we asked if they prefer to have an answer to their call at the time of the call or have a physician call them back, most stated they would rather have the answer when they call as long as they had confidence that the person was communicating with the physician. This explains why telephone nurse advice lines are so popular.

The reason physicians and patients alike become dependent on one person is because that is the one person who can answer their questions or solve their immediate problems. Systems need to be so clear as to appear seamless to patients when they interact with anyone in the office.

When staff members form a team and when roles, expectations and desired outcomes are clearly defined and agreed upon, a practice will function like a winning team. To make this happen, everyone needs to agree on how it is done.

First, recognize that it is probably impractical for every physician to have his or her own exclusive support staff. One-on-one staffing is not efficient unless you move all desk work to the front office.

Second, because staff will serve several different physicians, it is critical to establish uniform systems, routines and ongoing communications.

Third, craft each position carefully to include responsibilities that use the expertise of one of the three job categories: clerk, medical assistant and registered nurse. You must give your team a sense of purpose, control and realistic expectations.

You can further guide your team by clearly communicating the practice's mission statement. A mission statement outlines the goals of the practice. Place this statement where both staff members and patients can see it.

To help the team function as a single unit, you must develop communication tools.

Communication tools

There are three communication tools we recommend for every practice.

The first is the appointment schedule. Do not view the schedule as a tool for scheduling patients' appointments only. You also should view the schedule as a communication tool. It allows the scheduler to communicate with the back office staff member. The three major elements are time, appointment type and remarks.

The time helps the office staff members plan their day. The appointment type is a clue as to the length of time of the visit. The remarks column becomes the most valuable information. Here is where the clues are as to what information needs to be ready for the visit as well as how to prepare the exam room. A sample of this form is on the next page.

The second tool is the patient visit worksheet. This tool is to communicate information to the physician. You can use this tool three different ways.

First, the support staff members use the tool during visit prep to record any missing information, whether outside records have arrived, allergies, medications and so on.

Second, staff members use the tool during rooming. By annotating the appropriate appointment type on the top of the form, the person rooming the patient knows exactly what kind of information they must gather when rooming the patient.

Third, the physicians use the form to dictate notes from while talking with patients. This is not part of the medical record, so it will remain in the office until the transcriptionist completes the dictation. By dictating from this form, physicians are able to dictate all essential information, including information the support staff usually write in the medical record. This will be especially important as we move to an electronic medical record.

A sample of this form is on page 79.

The third tool we use is a patient visit order sheet. Physicians use this tool to communicate withtheir patients and then the staff. An order sheet gives you the opportunity to review the orders with the patient and give them a copy to take with them. Patients appreciate having a copy of their orders.

Give the original to your staff to process. This way you do not have to wait until they are off the phone to

Appointment schedule

Time	Name	MRN	Age	Appointment type	Remarks
7:50	John Doe	123456	45	Con	Miller/OSR/4-94/dia-betic
8:50	Jane Doe	654321	22	BV	B031/sore throat/3 days
9:00	Sue Smith	456123	35	New	NPE/3-91/no problems
9:40	Bill Jones	123654	55	EV	RPE/4-93/diabetic

Patient visit worksheet

Clinic #:
Personal physician:

Patient name:
Daytime phone:

Reason for visit

| New ☐ | Complete 1,2,4,5 | BV ☐ | Complete 1,4,5 |
| Con ☐ | Complete 1,2,3,4,5 | EV ☐ | Complete 1,2,4,5 |

1. Vital signs:

HT   WT   BP   Temp   LMP

2. Recent tests:

Lab   EKG   Mammogram   Treadmill   Echo   Procto   Other X-ray

3. Outside records:

Films   Records

4. Medications

Name   Dose   Last refill   Last appointment

5. Allergies:

Notes:

orally give them the orders. This will cut down on mistakes as well as time.

The last purpose for this form is order verification. Place this form in a tickler file until all orders are completed. The tickler file allows your staff to follow up on all outstanding orders.

This form also communicates your desire for patient education and follow-up.

A sample patient visit order sheet follows on the next page.

Weekly meetings

It is important to conduct short weekly meetings. Many groups choose one day a week to have lunch together and talk about how to improve service to the patients. An informal environment helps make all players feel relaxed and comfortable — team building at its best! No white coats or name badges at the meetings, please!

At these weekly meetings, value each person equally for their insights, suggestions and ideas. This will empower your staff to work on ways to improve support to the physician/patient interaction and improve value as perceived by the patient.

In addition to weekly meetings, the group should meet for five minutes each morning to examine daily operational issues.

The role of the morning huddle

How do you keep the sense of teamwork and interdependency going once the practice is running? Schedule a daily huddle — a short, informal meeting of the physician and his support staff first thing in the morning. The purpose of this meeting is to proactively plan the day's activities. You should include:

Patient visit order sheet

Patient name:
Daytime phone:

Clinic #:
Personal physician:

Special needs:
Outside records

Financial counseling

Test results:
(vehicle for informing patient of test results)
Call patient
Form letter
Dictated letter
Date reported

Visit follow-up
(appointment category and time frame)
BV   EV

Tests:
(list the most common tests ordered)
Lab: Stat   Routine   ICD-9

Radiology:

Cardiology:

Health maintenance:

Educational materials:

Nursing instructions:

- old business. Review yesterday's schedule. This is very helpful if you have new support staff. Review what went well and what did not go well. Identify key patients for follow-up calls to check on their progress. This is a major patient satisfier;

- new business. Review today's schedule for issues that are likely to arise: patients with unusual needs, special tests that may be required, staffing issues that everyone should know about. This is an ideal time to communicate how the physician would like the staff to handle same day urgent patients. By communicating this early in the day, your support staff will not have to interrupt you to ask you where and when to add patients; and

- future business. Review tomorrow's schedule. Look for scheduling problems that could cause havoc tomorrow. This will give you time to fix the problems and a chance to prepare for tomorrow. This is a good time to identify and call chronic missed-appointment patients or people who are always late.

In multispecialty clinics, there likely is another element of the team: administrative staff members.

It is just as important to keep lines of communication open with administration as it is with your physicians and staff. This open communication will lead to a sense of partnership.

Unfortunately, this communication does not always happen. Administrators and physicians find themselves at odds. Administrators press management to decrease operational expenses and physicians to increase productivity. This results in tremendous frustration for both physicians and management.

It is essentially a matter of focus: administrators are interested in cutting expenses; physicians are being asked to increase revenues.

Keeping costs in line and patient counts up are both necessary for a successful practice. The answer comes in collaboration, not in conflict.

Newly formed medical practices, as well as existing groups, benefit from close, ongoing communication between all team members, including staff members, physicians and administrators.

Chapter 11

Allocating resources by volume of work

Resource allocation is a hot topic in group practices. Historically, groups have allocated resources by discipline. For example, a physician may have been allocated one office, two exam rooms and an office assistant. A physician's assistant may have been allocated less: one shared office, one exam room and no support staff. Hierarchy dictated resource allocation.

Today, resources are allocated differently. We now realize that volume of work is key to allocation of resources. Physicians who see high volumes of patients per day need more support staff and more space to maximize their productivity.

We also realize that allied health professionals need support commensurate to their volume of work. Just because they are not physicians does not mean they do not generate a great deal of work.

Using patient visit volumes is one measurement for support staff and space needs. Patient visits generate most but not all of the clinic's work.

Space and resources are becoming more expensive. One way to combat this increase is to better utilize both support staff and space. We already discussed the advantages of using team staffing. However, we also must consider sharing exam rooms.

To effectively share exam room space, try the following. Hang a form on the outside of each exam room. Every time a patient is put in an exam room, have the support staff record the time. When the patient leaves the room, again record the time. Subtract the time out from the time in to establish the room utilization time for each patient. Compile all the times each day for several weeks. You will be amazed at what a small percentage of time each exam room is actually used.

This brings us back to the concept of master schedules. Often times you can add another physician without adding space if you become creative and stagger or expand hours. This increases physician availability, a plus for patients. By extending the hours you can better meet the needs of your patients.

Before and after work are popular appointment times for working patients. Lunch hour also is popular; however, this only works when physicians run on time. Senior citizens seem to prefer daylight hours. Working the usual 9 a.m. to noon and 2 to 5 p.m. May hinder the physician's ability to maintain an adequate patient base.

Allocating resources by volume of work will allow you to better manage your expenses, resulting in decreased cost per visit.

Now that you have an understanding of the six guiding principles of practice management. Let's look at a smooth-running medical practice that embraces all of these principles.

Chapter 12

A smooth operation

Let's look back at the fictitious case and see how Ann Ackney handled her situation.

After losing all confidence in Dr. Frazzle, Ackney began seeing Dr. Smooth.

It is Monday morning and Ms. Ackney calls Dr. Smooth's office for an appointment. Mary, the receptionist, courteously answers the phone. Mary asks Ann pertinent questions to establish the reason for the appointment, as well as information that will allow Mary to schedule Ann for the correct amount of time. Patient-focused scheduling enables Mary to find time in the schedule for Ann. Mary schedules Ann for Wednesday at 4:30 p.m. Before hanging up, Mary verifies Ann's demographic information to ensure that the Medical Records Department pulls the correct chart. It also allows Mary the opportunity to review Ann's co-pay responsibility. This will alleviate patient embarrassment or surprise at the time of the appointment.

The staff in the Medical Records Department automatically pulls Ms. Ackney's chart and sends it to Dr. Smooth's office.

On Tuesday afternoon, Betty, the registered nurse for Dr. Smooth and his partner, prepares charts for the next day. She pulls Ann's chart and quickly scans it for accuracy and completeness. She assesses any preparation needs for the visit. Betty notices that Ms. Ackney's last mammogram report is not in the chart, so Betty pulls the result up on the computer, prints it off and places it on the chart for the physician.

Wednesday morning, Suzy, the other support staff person, takes a quick inventory of all exam rooms and stocks them. Stocking exam rooms identically makes it faster and easier for Suzy to restock. When Dr. Smooth arrives at the clinic Wednesday, Suzy reviews yesterday's, today's and tomorrow's schedules with him. Because Suzy is fairly new, they are reviewing yesterday's schedule to learn how they can better work together. Dr. Smooth also notes that two of his patients from yesterday could use a personal call from the nurse to follow-up on their conditions.

As Dr. Smooth looks over today's schedule, he notes that one of the patients on his schedule was admitted to the hospital last night. Suzy cancels the appointment, allowing time to schedule another patient. Dr. Smooth also notes his 1 p.m. patient often forgets appointments and asks Suzy to call him.

As Dr. Smooth looks over tomorrow's schedule, he notes an error in the schedule. By correcting it today, they have alleviated confusion tomorrow as well as saved time. Reacting to a problem always takes more time than planning ahead. This entire process took less than five minutes, yet it alleviated confusion, a potentially missed appointment and inappropriate appointments and it facilitated appropriate follow-up on appropriate patients.

On Wednesday at 4:30 p.m., Ms. Ackney arrives and Mary greets her warmly. She notes there were no glass windows separating her from the receptionist. It feels much friendlier than Dr. Frazzle's office. After a quick check-in and payment of her co-pay, Ms. Ackney takes a seat in the clean, neat waiting room. Within five minutes Suzy walks up to Ms. Ackney and calls her by name. Ann responds and the two walk to the back office. On the way back, Suzy verifies Ms. Ackney's address and phone number to facilitate timely follow-up.

Because Ann is in for a chief complaint, Suzy takes her vital signs, identifies the medications she is presently taking and asks if she needs any refills. Suzy also asks about allergies, symptoms and duration of her chief complaint. Suzy completes part of the prescription for the medication Ann requests. She then records the information on the visit prep sheet and places it on the front of the chart. After instructing Ann to put on a gown, Suzy leaves the room, places the chart outside the door and marks the room number on the schedule hanging on Dr. Smooth's office door.

Five minutes later, Dr. Smooth completes dictating the last patient's chart and notes on his schedule that Ann is ready in room 22. Before Dr. Smooth enters the exam room, he sees a message on the clip between his exam rooms. He quickly glances at the message, noting it only needs a signature. After Dr. Smooth signs the message, drops it in the "out" box, he begins to review Ann's visit prep sheet and summary sheet on the front of Ann's chart. It takes less than two minutes to become familiar with Ann.

Dr. Smooth walks into the room and greets Ms. Ackney. He reviews her history with her and notes that the chart is accurate and complete. After concluding that Ann indeed needs the medication she is requesting, Dr. Smooth adjusts the dosage and signs the prescription Suzy prepared.

He decides to do a small procedure and notes everything he needs is in place. When he completes the exam, Dr. Smooth reviews the orders with Ann, discusses how Betty will call her tomorrow with the test results and hands Ann her prescription. Dr. Smooth then asks if she has any other questions. Ann feels relieved by the attention Dr. Smooth shows her and feels he is extremely competent, thorough and informative. She has no other questions. As Dr. Smooth leaves the exam room, he instructs Ms. Ackney to talk to Betty before she leaves the office.

When he walks back to his office to dictate, he hands Betty the order sheet. On the order sheet he requests educational materials for Ann and asks Betty to review the information with Ann. When he completes his dictation, he moves on to his last patient of the day. Once Dr. Smooth finishes his last patient, he returns to his office, dictates the last chart and prepares to leave. He glances in his action box and notes two forms to sign. Suzy places all action items in the "action" box with the appropriate back-up material attached. Since all the information he needs is available, he reviews each item and signs both. He then places them in his "out" box. He also quickly reviews the messages the nurse responded to today. Betty handled all calls appropriately; however, Dr. Smooth feels one of the calls needs follow-up tomorrow. He quickly jots a note to the nurse, places it in his "out" box and is off to make rounds in the hospital. It was another rewarding day for Dr. Smooth. He was able to care for 25 patients and still was out on time.

Meanwhile, Betty greets Ms. Ackney as she walks out of the exam room. Betty gives her some educational material and reviews it with her before she leaves. She also reviews the orders and gives Ann a copy to take with her in case she forgets what Dr. Smooth ordered. She then asks if Ann has any questions. Betty instructs Ann to stop by the lab on her way out of the clinic. They discuss an appropriate time for Betty to call with the results. Betty notes the time on the order sheet and places a copy of the order sheet in her tickler file.

The lab information is on the computer when Betty arrives at work Thursday morning. The lab values are slightly elevated; however, Betty knows from the prewritten orders how to handle the situation. At 1 p.m. Betty calls Ms. Ackney to give her the results of the lab tests and explain the plan of care. She documents her conversation with Ann. Dr. Smooth receives a copy of the documentation so he can better manage the care of his patients.

Ann is amazed when she receives a follow-up call from Betty on Friday, just to see how she is doing.

Dr. Smooth's efficient practice impresses Ann; it seems to run like clock work. When friends or acquaintances mention they are looking for a physician, Ann does not hesitate to refer Dr. Smooth.

Following the six guiding principles can transform a chaotic practice into a smooth-running operation. Energy is spent on productive activities. Physicians and staff complete more work in less time when they take the time to plan ahead.

Chapter 13

Tying it all together

You now know the basics of building a smooth-running, efficient practice. These principles will lead to an environment where patients are happy, because meeting their needs is the cornerstone of every activity.

Staff will enjoy stability, order, structure and freedom from fighting "fires." Finally, the physician's time will be used wisely. So, do you remember the elements of the efficient practice?

Review the key principles. As you do, do not just read them. Instead, think of how you can apply them.

Customer service

Build an efficient practice around the needs of the patient. Convenient hours, courteous service, thorough explanation of tests, timely follow-up, respect of privacy and becoming proactive guardians of that patient's health and well-being all reflect positive customer service.

Barrier-free practices

The efficient practice is barrier free. In a literal sense, that means that frosted glass windows are not pulled to separate the receptionist staff from the waiting room. However, it extends to removing other barriers such as always being there for the patient. When the patient needs help and information, someone is there. It does not always have to be a physician. It means supplying information when the patient needs it and having adequate backup so a patient feels cared for at all times.

Rules-based appointment types

In efficient practices, deciding how much time to book for an appointment is not a matter of guesswork. Instead, specific appointment lengths and types emerge from a series of carefully crafted triage questions. This helps assure that the time booked for a patient will be long enough to meet the patient's needs, without leaving the patient or physician feeling rushed. However, it is equally important that the time is not so long that you waste valuable physician time.

Knowledge and training for appropriate scheduling

If a physician's time is the basic building block of a practice, then the person who puts those blocks together is the builder of the office's profitability. The scheduler plays a vital function. While the rules-based appointment types provide the structure for a well-timed practice, it takes a knowledgeable, trained staff to make the plan work.

Invest in staff training.

Avoiding rework

Another way of saying this is, "Do it right the first time." This is important throughout the entire practice, but the attention to detail starts at the beginning of the practice. Collect complete and accurate information. Skilled staff should clarify answers, restate numbers, verify insurance coverage and collect the appropriate information. Starting out with a clean chart and accurate information builds credibility for the practice, shows patients a genuine concern and prevents the need to correct needless mistakes in the future.

Making a physician productive

Policies and structure should help doctors work smart, not hard. To do this, only physicians should do tasks that only they can do safely. Remember the axiom: "If you can safely and legally delegate downward, do it."

Staff members can do many tasks to save physicians time: review charts in advance, identify a patient's chief complaint, take vital signs, stock exam rooms appropriately, etc.

These steps mean that the physician can walk into the exam room, greet the patient by name, focus on the presenting complaint, complete the exam, develop the treatment plan, complete the order sheet and provide resource materials without scurrying around.

The physician is not distracted with needless details, so he or she can provide the single most important patient criteria for a good visit, "The doctor really listened to me."

Following every visit, the physician should immediately complete any necessary dictation, including treatment provided, future treatment plans and the need for follow-up, if any.

There is no better time to complete whatever initial documentation that insurance companies may require if a physician must complete it. The rule: do not procrastinate; get it done right away.

Holding a morning huddle

The staff should meet for a few minutes every day. The daily agenda is simple and includes three items:

- Is there any follow-up work from yesterday that needs to be completed?

- Are there any anticipated problems or challenges in today's schedule? and

- Are there any problems with tomorrow's schedule that need to be corrected today?

This daily get-together is a great way to quickly share information with the entire staff, thank people for extra effort, answer questions and discuss concerns.

Make communication routine and painless

Every day physicians and staff must process dozens of items of information. Good systems can make this happen efficiently. Evaluate the speed of response, the best person to respond and use the systems outlined in this book.

The underlying concepts

Years of experience go into building an efficient practice, as well as several key concepts, which are worth remembering.

Decisions made from data always are better than actions based on hunches

One piece of information does not establish a trend. One fact is not all you need to know; nor is one anecdote the whole story.

People running the most successful practices today make decisions based on solid information, collected over time, analyzed carefully and responded to with well-crafted solutions.

If you want to know what your customers want, simply ask them

Put the patients in charge of the practice. Ask them what they want. When they call with questions, ask, "How soon should we get back to you?" When they call to schedule an appointment, ask, "Is this time convenient with you...are we scheduling you soon enough?"

If you ask them, patients will be your strongest allies in building a practice that genuinely meets their needs. More importantly, if you listen and act on what a patient tells you, you will build loyalty that will last a lifetime.

Make all office functions support the core practice

At its core, a medical practice is about a physician spending time with a patient. Every activity and process should be aimed at making that encounter go smoothly, easily and successfully for both the physician and the patient.

If you peel off the many layers of a practice, this is the pearl that you will find at the center — physicians enjoying seeing patients.

Take the team approach

It is not a good use of a physician's time to stock exam rooms. Similarly, it does not make sense for a receptionist to give out medical advice.

As mentioned throughout this book, the litmus test of appropriateness is this: delegate tasks to the lowest skill level person who can do the task safely, legally and with credibility.

Efficient practices give great customer service

From the moment a person calls an efficiently and effectively run practice, it is immediately apparent that the practice values customer service. The receptionist quickly responds to the person by name, listens attentively, responds with concern and strives to accommodate the caller's wishes.

A new patient will experience that sense of service throughout his or her visit. Wait times will be reasonable. The time with the physician will be focused, attentive and informative. Follow-up communication will be timely, understandable and warm.

In an efficient practice you treat every patient like a first-class honored customer.

Make things uniform; strive for standardization

The physicians in a practice should decide what protocols, standards, vendors and supplies they want to use and stick to it. Variation creates waste. The need for more money in inventory, duplicate training and systems that may not be integrated is costly. The more variation there is, the less support physicians feel. Variation creates more complex systems that result in increased errors, inefficiencies and rework. If there is only one physician, obviously there is only one standard. When two physicians work together, it becomes more complex.

By the time you have 10 or more physicians, variation for each of them can cause absolute chaos within a practice.

One practice cut the costs of cataract surgery by 40 percent, simply by agreeing to use the same supplies, then negotiating a good price from the supplier.

The rule: establish one way of doing things and stick to it unless the group decides to change.

As simple and straightforward as these guidelines seem, they are seldom followed by most practices.

When you put these principles in place, a practice invariably runs much smoother, increases patient satisfaction, leads to more productive and happy physicians and staff and adds to the practice's profitability.

We encourage you to put these recommendations to the test in your own organization. The results will delight you.